BEST CROCK POT RECIPES 2021

SLOW COOKING RECIPES FOR ANY OCCASION

DELPHINE DALBERT

Table of Contents

Slow Cooker Lemon Chicken

INGREDIENTS

- 1 broiler-fryer,cut up, or about 3 1/2 pounds chicken pieces

- 1 teaspoon crumbled dry leaf oregano

- 2 cloves garlic, minced

- 2 tablespoons butter

- 1/4 cup dry wine, sherry, chicken broth, or water

- 3 tablespoons lemon juice

- Salt and pepper

PREPARATION

1. Season the chicken pieces with salt and pepper. Sprinkle half of garlic and oregano over the chicken.
2. Melt butter in a sauté pan over medium heat and brown chicken on all sides.
3. Transfer chicken to crockpot. Sprinkle with remaining oregano and garlic. Add wine or sherry to the sauté pan and stir to loosen brown bits; pour into slow cooker.
4. Cover and cook on LOW (200°) for 7 to 8 hours. Add lemon juice last hour.
5. Skim fat from juices and pour to a serving bowl; thicken juices, if desired.

6. Serve chicken with juices.
7. Serves 4.

Slow Cooker Stuffed Chicken Breasts
INGREDIENTS

-
6 boneless chicken breast halves, without skin

-
6 thin slices ham

-
6 thin slices Swiss cheese

-
1/2 cup all-purpose flour, seasoned with 1/2 teaspoon

-
salt and a dash of pepper

-
8 ounces fresh sliced mushrooms

-
1/2 cup chicken broth

-
1/2 cup dry white wine or Marsala

-
1/4 teaspoon ground rosemary

-
1/4 cup grated Parmesan cheese

-
2 teaspoons cornstarch

-
1 tablespoon cold water

- salt and pepper to taste

PREPARATION

1. Place chicken pieces between 2 pieces of waxed paper or plastic wrap and pound gently until evenly flattened. Place 1 slice of ham and 1 slice of cheese on each chicken breast; roll up and secure with toothpicks then roll in the seasoned flour. Put mushrooms in the crockpot and place chicken rolls on top of mushrooms. In a separate bowl, combine chicken broth, wine and rosemary; pour over chicken.
2. Sprinkle with the Parmesan cheese. Cover and cook on LOW for 6 hours. Just before serving, combine cornstarch and water. Remove chicken; add cornstarch mixture and stir until thickened. Add salt and paper to taste. Pour sauce over chicken and serve.
3. **Serves 6.**

Slow-Cooked Chicken Dijon

INGREDIENTS

- 1 to 2 pounds chicken breast tenders

- 1 can condensed cream of chicken soup, undiluted (10 1/2 ounce)

- 2 tablespoons regular or grainy Dijon mustard

- 1 tablespoon cornstarch

- 1/2 cup water

- pepper to taste

- 1 teaspoon dried parsley flakes or 1 tablespoon fresh chopped parsley

PREPARATION

1. Wash chicken and pat dry; arrange in the slow cooker. Combine the soup with mustard and cornstar; add water and stir. Stir in parsley and pepper. Pour the mixture over the chicken. Cover and cook on LOW for 6 to 7 hours. Serve with hot cooked rice and a side vegetable.
2. Chicken Dijon recipe serves 4 to 6.

Spanish Chicken with Olives and Tomatoes

INGREDIENTS

-
6 boneless chicken breast halves, skin removed

-
seasoned salt & pepper to taste

-
sliced ripe olives, 4 ounces

-
1 can (4 ounces) sliced mushrooms, drained

-
1 can (14.5 ounces) stewed tomatoes

-
Liquid to cover

-
(beer, tomato soup or tomato sauce w/equal amount of water or stock)

PREPARATION

1. Cut chicken breasts into bite-sized pieces; season. Combine with remaining ingredients in slow cooker. Cover and cook on LOW for 5 to 7 hours. Serve with hot cooked rice.
2. Serves 4 to 6.

Spicy Crockpot Chicken With Chipotle Marmalade Sauce

INGREDIENTS

- 1 chipotle pepper in adobo sauce, finely chopped, with about 1 teaspoon of the sauce

- 1/3 cup sweet orange marmalade

- 1 teaspoon chili powder

- 1/4 teaspoon garlic powder

- 1 tablespoon balsamic vinegar

- 1 tablespoon honey

- 1/2 cup chicken broth

- 1 tablespoon vegetable oil

- Dash freshly ground black pepper

- Dash salt

- 4 boneless chicken breast halves, without skin

-

1 tablespoon cornstarch

-

2 tablespoons cold water

PREPARATION

1. Combine the chipotle with adobo sauce, marmalade, chili powder, garlic powder, vinegar, honey, chicken broth, and oil.
2. Sprinkle the chicken breasts with salt and pepper. Arrange them in the slow cooker; pour marmalade mixture over all.
3. Cover and cook on LOW for 5 to 7 hours, or until chicken is cooked through.
4. Put the chicken on a plate; cover and keep warm.
5. Pour the liquids into a saucepan and bring to a boil over high heat.
6. Reduce heat to medium and boil until slightly reduced, about 5 minutes.
7. Combine the cornstarch with cold water until smooth; stir into the sauce and continue cooking, stirring, for about 1 minute longer, or until thickened.
8. Serve the chicken with the thickened sauce.
9. Serves 4.
10. The recipe can be doubled and cooked for the same amount of time.

Swiss Chicken Casserole Recipe, Crock Pot

INGREDIENTS

- 6 boneless chicken breast halves, skin removed

- 6 slices Swiss cheese

- 1 can condensed (10 3/4 ounces) cream of mushroom soup, undiluted

- 2 cups herb-seasoned stuffing mix

- 1/2 cup butter or margarine, melted

PREPARATION

1. Butter the sides and bottom of the crockery insert of the slow cooker or spray with nonstick cooking spray.
2. Arrange the chicken breasts in the bottom of the pot. Top with the Swiss cheese and then spoon the cream of mushroom soup over cheese.
3. Sprinkle the stuffing crumbs over the soup layer and then drizzle melted butter over the top.
4. Cook on LOW for 5 to 7 hours or high 3 to 3 1/2 hours.

Tami's Honey-Mustard Chicken

INGREDIENTS

- 4 to 6 boneless skinless chicken breast halves (or use other pieces of chicken)

- 3/4 cup Dijon mustard or use a favorite gourmet mustard

- 1/4 cup honey

PREPARATION

1. Put chicken in pot. Mix mustard and honey and pour over chicken. Cook on high for 3 hours or on low for 6 to 8 hours. Adjust time for bone-in chicken.

Tami's Lemon Pepper Chicken, Slow Cooker

INGREDIENTS

- 4 to 6 boneless chicken breast halves, skin removed, or other chicken parts

- lemon pepper seasoning

- 2 tablespoons melted butter or margarine

PREPARATION

1. Put chicken in slow cooker. Sprinkle generously with lemon pepper seasoning. Drizzle butter or margarine over chicken. Cook on LOW for 6 to 8 hours, or until chicken is tender.

Tawny's Crock \"Pop\" Chicken

INGREDIENTS

- 1 1/2 to 2 1/2 pounds chicken pieces, breasts, etc.

- 1 small bottle ketchup (1 cup)

- 1 medium onion, chopped

- 1 can your favorite brand of cola, or Dr. Pepper®

PREPARATION

1. Combine all ingredients in the slow cooker; cover and cook on low for 6 to 8 hours.
2. Serve over rice, noodles, or potatoes.
3. Serves 4 to 6.

White Chili With Chicken

INGREDIENTS

-
1 can cooking oil spray

-
1 tablespoon olive oil

-
1 pound boneless chicken breast; skin removed, cut in 1/2-inch pieces

-
1/4 cup chopped onion

-
3 cloves garlic, minced

-
1 can tomatillos (about 16 ounces), drained and cut up

-
1 can Ro-tel tomatoes, diced tomatoes with green chiles

-
1 can chicken broth (1 1/2 cups)

-
1 can (4 ounces) chopped green chile peppers, not drained

-
1/2 teaspoon dried oregano flakes

-
1/2 teaspoon coriander seeds, crushed

-
1/4 teaspoon ground cumin

- 2 cans great northern beans, drained

- 3 tablespoons lime juice

- 1/4 teaspoon black pepper

- 1/2 cup shredded sharp Cheddar cheese

PREPARATION

1. Spray a large skillet with cooking spray, add olive oil and heat on medium high until hot. Add diced chicken and saute for 3 minutes or until done. Remove chicken from pan. Place all ingredients, except Cheese, in a crockpot and cook for 8 hours. Top each serving with a little shredded cheese. Serve white chicken chili with tortilla chips, salsa, sour cream, and condiments of your choice. Serves 6 .

Will's Chicken Chili for the Slow Cooker

INGREDIENTS

- 1 pound chicken breast halves or tenders

- 2 cans (approx. 14.5 oz. each) chicken broth

- 2 cans (8 oz. each) cans tomato sauce

- 1 onion, diced

- 1 cup frozen corn

- 1 carrot, sliced

- 1 celery stalk, diced

- 1 can (14.5 ounces) can diced tomatoes

- 1 15-ounce can red kidney beans, plus liquid

- 1 jar (4 ounces) diced pimiento, drained

- 1 jalapeno pepper, diced

- 2 teaspoons chili powder (or more to taste)

- 1 teaspoon cumin

- 1 clove garlic, minced (can substitute garlic powder)

- 1/2 teaspoon salt

- dash basil

- dash cayenne pepper (or more to taste)

- dash oregano

-

optional garnishes

- sour cream

- minced parsley

- shredded cheese (Mexican blend, cheddar jack, cheddar, pepper jack, etc.)

- diced tomatoes

- thinly sliced green onions

PREPARATION

1. Combine all ingredients except optional garnishes in the slow cooker. Cover and cook on high for 2 hours, then low for 6 additional hours.
2. Or the chili can be cooked on low for 8 to 10 hours.
3. Serve in bowls with your choice of garnishes.

Chunky Turkey Chili

INGREDIENTS

- 1 pound ground turkey or ground beef

- 1/2 cup coarsely chopped onion

- 2 cans (14.5 ounces each) diced tomatoes with juice

- 1 can (16 ounces) pinto beans, drained, rinsed

- 1/2 cup chunky salsa, your favorite

- 2 teaspoons chili powder

- 1 1/2 teaspoons ground cumin

- salt and pepper to taste

- 1/2 cup shredded Cheddar or Mexican blend cheese

- 1 to 2 tablespoons sliced black olives

PREPARATION

1. In a large skillet over medium heat, brown ground turkey and onion. Drain off excess fat.
2. Transfer browned mixture to the crockpot with tomatoes, beans, salsa, chili powder, and cumin. Stir gently to blend ingredients.
3. Cover and cook on LOW setting for 5 to 6 hours. Taste and season with salt and pepper.
4. Serve with a dollop of sour cream and a little shredded cheese and black olive slices.
5.

Serves 4.

Cranberry-Apple Turkey Breast

INGREDIENTS

- 2 tablespoons butter

- 1 large rib celery, chopped

- 2 tablespoons finely chopped onion or shallot, optional

- 1 apple, peeled, cored, and diced

- 2 cups herb-seasoned stuffing crumbs

- 1/2 cup chicken broth

- 1 can (14 ounces) whole berry cranberry sauce, divided

- 1 teaspoon poultry seasoning

- turkey breast cutlets, about 1 1/2 to 2 pounds

- kosher salt and freshly ground black pepper

PREPARATION

1. In a large skillet or saute pan over medium heat, melt the butter. Add the celery, onion, if using, and the diced apple. Cook, stirring, for about 5 minutes.
2. In a large bowl, combine the stuffing crumbs with the sauteed vegetable mixture, chicken broth, 1 cup of the cranberry sauce, and the poultry seasoning. Mix well to blend.
3. Spoon a few tablespoons of stuffing mixture on a turkey breast cutlet. Starting with the long end roll up and secure with toothpicks.
4. Arrange the rolls in the slow cooker.
5. Alternatively, you can lightly roll the turkey up without the stuffing and spoon the stuffing mixture around the rolls.
6. Spoon any excess stuffing mixture around the turkey rolls. Sprinkle with kosher salt and freshly ground black pepper.
7. Cover and cook on LOW for 5 hours, or on HIGH for about 2 1/2 hours.

Turkey Breast with Orange Cranberry Sauce

INGREDIENTS

- 1/4 cup granulated sugar

- 2 tablespoons cornstarch

- 3/4 cup orange marmalade

- 1 cup fresh cranberries, ground or finely chopped

- 1 small boneless turkey breast, about 3 to 4 pounds

- salt and pepper to taste

PREPARATION

1. In small saucepan, blend sugar and cornstarch; stir in marmalade and cranberries. Cook over medium heat, stirring, until mixture is bubbly and slightly thickened.
2. Place turkey breast in slow cooker. Sprinkle all over with salt and pepper.
3. Pour the sauce over turkey.
4. Cover and cook on HIGH for 1 hour. Reduce heat to LOW and cook 6 to 8 hours longer.
5. Insert an instant-read thermometer into the thickest part of the turkey breast to check for doneness.
6. It should register at least 165° F to 170° F.
7. Slice turkey and serve with sauce.
8. Makes 6 to 8 servings.

Cranberry Turkey in a Crockpot

INGREDIENTS

-
1 turkey breast, thawed in refrigerator

-
1 envelope Lipton onion soup mix (I used the herb one)

-
1 can cranberry sauce

PREPARATION

1. Place the turkey in the Crock Pot. Mix together cranberry sauce and soup mix and pour over turkey.
2. Cook on high for 2 hours, then on low for 6 to 7 hours.
3. The turkey breast should register at least 165 on a food thermometer inserted in the thickest part of the meat.

Crockpot Turkey With Sour Cream

INGREDIENTS

- 1 boneless breast of turkey (about 3 1/2 pounds)

- 1 teaspoon salt

- 1/4 teaspoon pepper

- 2 teaspoons dried dillweed, divided

- 1/4 cup water

- 1 tablespoon white or wine vinegar

- 3 tablespoons flour

- 1 cup sour cream

PREPARATION

1. Sprinkle both sides of turkey breast with salt, pepper and 1 teaspoon dillweed. Place turkey breast in crockpot. Add water and vinegar. Cover and cook on low for 7 to 9 hours or until tender. Remove turkey breast to a platter; keep warm. Transfer juices to a saucepan; place on stovetop and heat over medium-high heat. Let simmer briskly, uncovered, for about 5 minutes to reduce the liquids. Dissolve flour in small amount of cold water and stir into the liquid.
2. Add the remaining teaspoon of dill weed.
3. Cook on until thickened, about 15 to 20 minutes. Stir in sour cream and turn off heat. Slice meat and serve with the sour cream sauce.
4. Serves 6.

Turkey Sandwiches

INGREDIENTS

- 6 c. diced turkey

- 3 cups Velveeta cheese (American cheese), diced or shredded

- 1 can (10 3/4 ounces) cream of mushroom soup

- 1 can (10 3/4 ounces) cream of chicken soup

- 1 onion, chopped

- 1/2 c. Miracle Whip

PREPARATION

1. In slow cooker, mix together diced turkey, cheese, cream of mushroom soup, cream of chicken soup, onion, and Miracle Whip. Cover and cook on low for 3 to 4 hours. Stir turkey mixture occasionally. Add a little water, if needed. Serve with split buns.

Crockpot Turkey With Garlic

INGREDIENTS

- 1 1/2 pounds boneless turkey thighs, skin removed

- salt and pepper or lemon pepper to taste

- 1 tablespoon olive oil

- 6 cloves garlic, left whole

- 1/2 cup dry white wine

- 1/2 cup chicken broth

- 1 tablespoon chopped parsley

PREPARATION

1. Season turkey with salt and pepper or lemon pepper. In a large skillet over medium-high heat, heat olive oil. Add turkey thighs; brown for about 10 minutes.
2. Place turkey in slow cooker; add remaining ingredients. Cook on HIGH for 3 to 4 hours, or until turkey thighs are cooked through. Remove garlic cloves from pot. Mash a few and return to the slow cooker, if desired. Serve turkey with juices.
3. Serves 4 to 6.

Ground Turkey Pasta Sauce

INGREDIENTS

- 3 tablespoons olive oil

- 1 lb. ground turkey

- 1 (14.5 oz.) can of stewed tomatoes

- 1 (6 oz.) can tomato paste

- 1/2 tsp. dry thyme

- 1 teaspoon dried leaf basil

- 1/2 tsp. oregano

- 1/2 to 1 teaspoon sugar, optional

- 1 teaspoon salt, or to taste

- 1/2 cup chopped onion

- 1 bell pepper, chopped

- 2 cloves crushed garlic

-

1 bay leaf

-

1/4 cup water

-

4 ounces chopped or sliced mushrooms, fresh or canned drained

PREPARATION

1. Put oil in skillet; brown ground turkey slowly. While ground turkey is cooking, put stewed tomatoes, tomato paste, thyme, basil, oregano, salt and sugar in slow cooker. Stir well and cook on low heat. When turkey is browned, transfer to slow cooker with slotted spoon. In pan drippings, sauté onion, pepper, garlic, and bay leaf until softened. To slow cooker, add 1/4 cup of water and the chopped mushrooms.
2. Cover and cook on low 4 to 6 hours. Thin with a little water if necessary.
3. Serve with hot cooked spaghetti your favorite cooked pasta.
4. Serves 6.

Ground Turkey Sloppy Joes

INGREDIENTS

- 2 pounds ground turkey

- 1 cup chopped onion

- 2 cans (15 oz each) tomato sauce

- 1 can (6 oz) tomato paste

- 1/2 cup brown sugar (firmly packed)

- 1/3 cup red wine or cider vinegar

- 2 tablespoons Worcestershire sauce

- 2 tablespoons liquid smoke

- 1/2 teaspoon seasoned salt

- 1/4 teaspoon black pepper

PREPARATION

1. Brown turkey with onions over medium-high heat about 6 to 8 minutes. Drain.
2. Transfer the turkey and onions to slow cooker. Stir in the remaining ingredients.
3. Cover and cook on low 6 to 7 hours. Serve on rolls or sliced bread.
4. Serves 8 to 10.

Easy Slow Cooker Cassoulet
INGREDIENTS

-
1 tablespoon extra virgin olive oil

-
1 large onion, finely chopped

-
4 boneless skinless chicken thighs, coarsely chopped

-
1/4 pound cooked smoked sausage, such as kielbasa or spicier andouille, diced

-
3 cloves garlic, minced

-
1 teaspoon dried thyme leaves

-
1/2 teaspoon black pepper

-
4 tablespoons tomato paste

-
2 tablespoons water

-
3 cans (about 15 ounces each) great northern beans, rinsed and drained

-
3 tablespoons chopped fresh parsley

PREPARATION

1. Heat olive oil in large skillet over medium heat.
2. Add onion to hot oil and cook, stirring, until onion is tender, about 4 minutes.
3. Stir in chicken, sausage, garlic, thyme, and pepper. Cook 5 to 8 minutes, or until chicken and sausage are browned.
4. Stir in tomato paste and water; transfer to slow cooker. Stir great northern beans into the chicken mixture; cover and cook on LOW for 4 to 6 hours.
5. Before serving, sprinkle the chopped parsley over cassoulet.
6. Serves 6.

Island Barbecued Turkey Legs

INGREDIENTS

- 4 to 6 turkey legs

- Salt and pepper

- 1/2 cup ketchup

- 5 tablespoons cider vinegar

- 1 tablespoon Worcestershire sauce

- 4 tablespoons dark brown sugar

- 1 teaspoon liquid smoke, optional

- 1 can (8 ounces) crushed pineapple, well drained

- 1/2 cup chopped onion

PREPARATION

1. Lightly grease the crockery liner of the slow cooker. Arrange the turkey legs in the slow cooker and sprinkle with salt and pepper. Combine the remaining ingredients; spoon over the turkey legs and turn to coat legs well. Cover and cook on LOW for 7 to 9 hours.

2. Serves 4 to 6.

Lemon Herb Turkey Breast

INGREDIENTS

- 1/4 cup granulated sugar

- 2 tablespoons cornstarch

- 3/4 cup orange marmalade

- 1 cup fresh cranberries, ground or finely chopped

- 1 small boneless turkey breast, about 3 to 4 pounds

- salt and pepper to taste

PREPARATION

1. In small saucepan, blend sugar and cornstarch; stir in marmalade and cranberries. Cook over medium heat, stirring, until mixture is bubbly and slightly thickened.
2. Place turkey breast in slow cooker. Sprinkle all over with salt and pepper.
3. Pour the sauce over turkey.
4. Cover and cook on HIGH for 1 hour. Reduce heat to LOW and cook 6 to 8 hours longer.
5. Insert an instant-read thermometer into the thickest part of the turkey breast to check for doneness.
6. It should register at least 165° F to 170° F.
7. Slice turkey and serve with sauce.
8. Makes 6 to 8 servings.

Slow Cooker Turkey and Wild Rice

INGREDIENTS

- 6 to 8 slices bacon, diced, fried until crisp and drained

- 1 pound turkey tenderloins, cut into 1-inch pieces

- 1/2 cup chopped onion

- 1/2 cup sliced carrots

- 1/2 cup sliced celery

- 2 cans (14 1/2 oz. each) chicken

- broth, or 3 1/4 cups of broth made from base or granules

- 1 can (10 3/4 oz). condensed cream of chicken soup or cream of chicken soup with herbs

- 1/4 tsp. dried marjoram

- 1/8 tsp. pepper

- 1 1/4 cups uncooked wild rice, rinsed

PREPARATION

1. In a heavy skillet, cook bacon until crispy; remove with slotted spoon and set aside. In drippings, brown the turkey pieces, cooking for about 3 to 4 minutes. Add onion, carrot, and celery; cook and stir 2 minutes.
2. Whisk together half of the broth and the soup in slow cooker. Stir in remaing broth, marjoram and the pepper. Stir in turkey mixture, bacon and the wild rice.
3. Cover and cook on high for 30 minutes.
4. Reduce heat to low. Cook 6-7 hours until rice is tender and liquid is absorbed. Turkey and wild rice serves 6.

Slow Cooked Turkey and Vegetables

INGREDIENTS

- boneless turkey breast, about 1 1/2 to 2 pounds

- 1 onion (cut into four slices)

- 2 small potatoes, sliced

- 2 small turnips, diced, optional

- baby carrots

- 1 package of dry chicken gravy mix

- 3/4 cup of dry white wine

- 1/4 cup water

PREPARATION

1. Season turkey with salt pepper and brown on all sides in skillet sprayed with cooking spray.
2. Add onion and cook until lightly browned.
3. Spray slow cooker with cooking spray and put carrots on the bottom; continue layering potatoes, turnips and onions.
4. Place turkey on top of vegetables.
5. Mix gravy with the wine and water; heat on stovetop or in microwave then pour over the turkey and vegetables.
6. Cover and cook on high for 2 hours and then turn to LOW and cook 3 to 4 hours longer.
7. Serves 4.

Turkey Breast Tenders with Orange-Cranberry Sauce

INGREDIENTS

- 2 lbs turkey breast tenders

- 1/3 cup orange juice

- 3/4 cup whole cranberry sauce

- 2 tablespoons brown sugar

- 1 tablespoon soy sauce

- 1/2 teaspoon allspice

- 1 tablespoon cornstarch dissolved in 1 tablespoon cold water

- salt and pepper to taste

PREPARATION

1. Combine all ingredients; turn turkey to coat. Cover and cook on low for 7 to 9 hours, or on high for 3 1/2 to 4 hours. About 10 minutes before serving, stir in the cornstarch/cold water mixture. Season to taste with salt and pepper.
2. Serves 4.

Turkey With Sweet Potatoes

INGREDIENTS

- 3 medium sweet potatoes or regular potatoes, peeled and cut into 2-inch cubes

- 1 1/2 to 2 pounds turkey thighs, skin removed

- 1 jar (12 ounces) turkey gravy (or use 1 1/2 to 2 cups)

- 2 tbsp. flour

- 1 tsp. dried parsley

- 1/2 teaspoon dried rosemary crushed

- 1/4 teaspoon dried leaf thyme

- 1/8 tsp. pepper

- 1 1/2 to 2 cups frozen cut green beans

PREPARATION

1. Layer sweet potatoes and turkey in slow cooker.
2. Combine gravy, flour, parsley, rosemary, thyme, and pepper; stir until smooth. Pour gravy mixture over the turkey and sweet potatoes.
3. Cover and cook on high for 1 hour. Reduce heat to low and cook 5 hours longer.
4. Add the green beans to the slow cooker; stir. Cover and cook 1 to 2 hours, or until turkey is tender and juices run clear.
5. Remove turkey and vegetables to a serving dish with a slotted spoon.
6. Stir sauce and serve with turkey and vegetables.
7. Serves 6

Crock Pot Turkey and Rice

INGREDIENTS

- 2 cans (10 3/4 ounces each) cream of mushroom soup or cream of celery soup

- 2 1/2 cups water

- 2 1/2 cups uncooked converted white rice

- 1 cup sliced celery

- 1/4 cup finely chopped onion

- 2 cups cubed cooked turkey

- 2 cups frozen peas and carrots

- 1 teaspoon poultry seasoning blend

PREPARATION

1. Pour soup and water into the slow cooker and mix to blend thoroughly. Add remaining ingredients and stir. Cook 5 to 7 hours on Low or 2 1/2 to 3 1/2 hours on High. Check from time to time to make sure rice does not get mushy. Serves 8.

Easy Slow Cooked Turkey Breast

INGREDIENTS

- 1 turkey breast, about 5 pounds

- 1/2 cup (4 ounces) melted butter

- salt and pepper

- 2 tablespoons cornstarch blended with 2 tablespoons water

- 1/2 to 1 cup chicken broth, as needed

PREPARATION

1. Sprinkle salt and pepper over the turkey breast and arrange in a large slow cooker. Pour melted butter over the turkey.
2. Cover and cook on HIGH for 6 to 7 hours, or until turkey gets brown and juices run clear when pierced with a knife.
3. Pour the juices from the slow cooker into a saucepan. Bring to boil slowly, then add cornstarch and water mixture. Add a little chicken broth, about 1/2 to 1 cup, depending on the amount of liquids left in the crockpot.
4. Whisk over medium-low heat until smooth and thickened.

Tamale Pie with Ground Turkey

INGREDIENTS

- 1 pound ground turkey

- 3/4 cup yellow cornmeal

- 1 1/2 cups milk

- 1 egg, beaten

- 1 package (1 1/4 ounce) chili seasoning mix

- 1 can (11 to 16 ounces) whole kernel corn, drained

- 1 can (14.5 to 16 ounces) tomatoes, cut up

- 1 cups shredded cheese

PREPARATION

1. Brown turkey and drain well. In bowl, mix cornmeal, milk and egg. Add drained meat, dry chili mix, tomatoes and corn. Stir. Pour into 3 1/2-quart or larger slow cooker. Cover and cook 1 hour on high, then turn to low and cook 3 hours on low. Sprinkle with cheese. Cook another 5 to 10 minutes.
2. Serves 6.

Turkey Barbecue

INGREDIENTS

- 2 to 3 pounds turkey cutlets or chops

- 2 green bell peppers, or combination of red, yellow, and green, cut in strips

- 1 teaspoon celery salt

- Dash of pepper

- 1 to 2 tablespoons finely chopped onion, or 2 teaspoons dried minced onion

- 2 cups thick barbecue sauce

PREPARATION

1. Sprinkle turkey cutlets with salt and pepper. Bake in 350° oven for 1 hour covered. Uncover for desired darker color. Meanwhile, combine barbecue sauce and celery salt in 5 quart slow cooker. Add green peppers and onions. Cover and cook on high while turkey is baking. Chop turkey (as desired in small to medium chunks) and add to slow cooker/Crock Pot. Cover and cook on low for 4 hours or HIGH for 2 hours.
2. Serve with fresh split rolls.
3. Turkey recipe serves 4 to 6.

Crockpot Turkey and Quesadillas

INGREDIENTS

-

1 turkey breast, about 5 pounds, bone-in

-

3/4 cup parsley, divided

-

1/2 cup vegetable oil

-

2 tablespoons salt

-

2 tablespoons black pepper

-

1 cup apple cider vinegar

PREPARATION

1. Place turkey in a large slow cooker. Stir together 1/2 cup of the chopped parsley, vegetable oil, salt, pepper and vinegar; pour over turkey breast. Sprinkle remaining parsley over top. Cook 4 to 4 1/2 hours on high or 8 to 9 hours on low. Remove from slow cooker and let stand 15 minutes before slicing.
2. Serves 6.
3. To make the Turkey Ouesadillas: Heat 1 teaspoon oil in a skillet over medium heat. Place a flour tortilla in the skillet and spread with about 1/2 cup of Mexican-style cheese blend and 1/4 to 1/2 cup diced turkey.
4. Top with a second tortilla. Cook until cheese starts to melt. Turn with a spatula and brown the other side. Cut quesadilla into quarters and serve with salsa.
5. Serves 6

Turkey Breast with Marmalade

INGREDIENTS

- turkey breast (to fit in crockpot)

- 1 jar orange marmalade or pineapple orange jam

- cinnamon

PREPARATION

1. Place a turkey breast in the slow cooker/Crock Pot, pour 1 jar Orange Marmalade or Pineapple/Orange Jam over the breast and sprinkle a little cinnamon on top. Cook on low for 6 to 8 hours or on high for about 4 hours.

Slow Cooker Turkey and Broccoli Casserole

INGREDIENTS

- 8 ounces mushrooms

- 2 tablespoons butter

- 1 can (10 3/4 ounces) condensed golden mushroom soup

- 5 tablespoons mayonnaise, about 1/3 cup

- 3 tablespoons milk

- 1 tablespoon prepared mustard

- 1/4 teaspoon black pepper

- 4 cups diced cooked turkey

- 16 ounces frozen cut broccoli

- 1 cup shredded American cheese

- 1/4 cup toasted almonds•, optional

PREPARATION

1. Spray inside of crockpot with cooking spray or lightly grease with butter.
2. In a skillet over medium low heat, sauté sliced mushrooms in butter until tender. In crockpot, combine mushrooms, soup, mayonnaise, milk, mustard, and pepper. Stir in diced turkey and broccoli. Cover and cook on LOW setting for 5 hours. Stir in cheese; cover and cook 30 minutes longer. Sprinkle with toasted almonds, if desired, just before serving.
3. Serves 6.

•To toast nuts, spread out in a single layer on a baking sheet. Toast in a 350° oven, stirring occasionally, for 10 to 15 minutes. Or, toast in an ungreased skillet over medium heat, stirring, until golden brown and aromatic.

Slow Cooker Turkey Pie

INGREDIENTS

- 3 cups diced cooked chicken or turkey

- 2 cans (14 1/2 ounce each) chicken broth

- 1/2 teaspoon salt

- 1/2 teaspoon pepper

- 1 stalk celery, thinly sliced

- 1/2 cup chopped onion

- 1 small bay leaf

- 3 cups cubed potatoes

- 1 package frozen mixed vegetables (16 oz)

- 1 cup milk

- 1 cup flour

- 1 teaspoon black pepper

-

1/2 teaspoon poultry seasoning blend

-

1/2 teaspoon salt

-

1 9-inch refrigerated pie crust

PREPARATION

1. Combine chicken, chicken broth, 1/2 teaspoon salt, 1/2 teaspoon pepper, celery, onion, bay leaf, potatoes, and mixed vegetables in slow cooker. Cover and cook on low 7 to 9 hours or on high 3 1/2 to 4 1/2 hours. Remove bay leaf.

2. Heat oven to 375°. In a small bowl, mix milk and flour. Gradually stir flour and milk mixture into the slow cooker. Stir in pepper, poultry seasoning, and salt. Remove the liner from slow cooker base and carefully place 9-inch pie crust over the mixture.

3. **Place the crockery inside pre-heated oven and bake (uncovered) for about 15 to 20 minutes, or until browned. If your liner is not removable or is too large for the crust, put the mixture in a casserole dish, cover with the pie crust and bake as above.**

4. Serves 8.

Turkey with Gravy

INGREDIENTS

- 1 to 1 1/2 pounds turkey breast tenders (cut in half if large), or sliced turkey cutlets

- 1 packet turkey gravy mix (dry)

- 1 can cream of mushroom soup (regular or 98% fat free)

- 1 tablespoon mushroom-onion soup mix (dry mix, about 1/2 packet), or use a few

- tablespoons of chopped onion and dry or canned mushrooms

- salt and pepper to taste

PREPARATION

1. Combine all ingredients in the Crock Pot; cover and cook on low for 6 1/2 to 8 hours. Serve with rice or potatoes.
2. Serves 4.

Turkey Madeira

INGREDIENTS

-
1 1/2 lb turkey breast tenders

-
2 ounces dried mushrooms

-
3/4 cup chicken broth

-
3 tablespoons Madeira wine

-
1 tablespoon lemon juice

-
salt and pepper to taste

PREPARATION

1. Cover and cook on low for 6 to 8 hours. Thicken juices with cornstarch if desired, and serve with rice.
2. Serves 4.

Ranch Turkey Thighs

INGREDIENTS

-
3 turkey thighs

-
Salt and pepper

-
1 envelope enchilada sauce mix

-
1 can (6 oz.) tomato paste

-
1/2 cup water

-
2 cup shredded Monterey Jack cheese

-
1/2 cup sour cream

-
1/4 cup chopped green onions

-
1 can (4 ounces) sliced ripe olives

PREPARATION

1. Cut each turkey thigh in half and remove the bone. Sprinkle the turkey with salt and pepper and arrange in the slow cooker insert.
2. Combine enchilada sauce mix, tomato paste, and water; stir until well blended. Spread the sauce mixture on top of turkey thighs.
3. Cover and cook on LOW for 6 to 7 hours, or until turkey is tender. Turn control to HIGH; stir in cheese and continue stirring until cheese is melted.
4. Transfer to a serving dish and top with sour cream and chopped green onions.
5. Garnish with sliced ripe olives.
6. Serve with tortillas and Easy Mexican Rice, if desired.
7. Serves 4 to 6.

Crockpot Turkey and Rice Casserole

INGREDIENTS

- 2 cans (10 3/4 ounces each) condensed cream of mushroom soup

- 3 cups water

- 3 cups converted long-grain white rice (uncooked)

- 1 cup thinly sliced celery

- 2 to 3 cups cubed cooked turkey

- 2 cups frozen mixed vegetables (peas & carrots, oriental mix, etc.)

- 1 teaspoon poultry seasoning

- 1 tablespoon dried minced onion

PREPARATION

1. Combine soup and water in slow cooker. Add remaining ingredients and mix well. Cover and cook 6 to 7 hours on low or about 3 to 3 1/2 hours on high, until rice is tender but not mushy.
2. Serves 4 to 6.

Turkey Stew with Mushrooms and Sour Cream

INGREDIENTS

-
1 pound turkey chops or cutlets, cut into 3- X 1-inch strips

-
1 medium onion, halved and thinly sliced

-
3 green onions with green, minced

-
8 ounces sliced fresh mushrooms

-
3 tablespoons all-purpose flour

-
1 cup milk or half-and-half

-
1 teaspoon dried leaf tarragon, crumbled

-
1 teaspoon dried parsley

-
1 teaspoon salt

-
1/8 teaspoon pepper

-
1/2 cup frozen peas and carrots

-
1/2 cup sour cream

PREPARATION

1. In a slow cooker, layer turkey strips, onions, and mushrooms. Cover and cook on LOW setting for 4 hours. Remove to a warm serving bowl then turn slow cooker to HIGH.
2. Combine flour and milk until flour is dissolved and mixture is smooth; stir into juices in slow cooker. Add tarragon, parsley, salt, and pepper. Return turkey and vegetables to the pot; add frozen vegetables. Cover and cook on HIGH for 1 hour, or until sauce is thickened and vegetables are done.
3. If desired, stir in sour cream just before serving. Serve over rice or toast points, if desired.
4. Serves 4.

Easy Crockpot Turkey Tetrazzini

INGREDIENTS

- 1 cup hot water

- 1 can (10 3/4-ounce) cream of chicken soup, or cream of chicken with herbs

- 1 can (4 ounces) mushrooms, with liquid

- 2 tablespoons chopped pimiento

- 2 cups diced cooked turkey

- 1 cup shredded Cheddar cheese

- 1/4 cup finely chopped onion

- 1 teaspoon dried parsley flakes

- dash nutmeg

- 2 cups broken uncooked spaghetti

PREPARATION

1. Spray inside of slow cooker crock with flavored cooking spray. In a bowl, combine the water, soup, mushrooms with liquid, and pimiento. Stir in the turkey, cheese, onion, parsley, and nutmeg. Add broken up spaghetti. Stir to combine and pour into crockpot. Cover and cook on LOW for 4 to 6 hours, until spaghetti is tender. Mix before serving. Serves 4 to 6.

Vickie's Spaghetti Sauce With Turkey Sausage

INGREDIENTS

- 6 ounces tomato paste

- 16 ounces stewed tomatoes

- 8 ounces tomato sauce

- 28 ounces tomatoes, canned, drained

- 1/2 cup red wine

- 1/2 cup water

- 1/2 teaspoon sugar

- 1/8 teaspoon dried leaf oregano

- 1/8 teaspoon dried leaf basil

- 1 bay leaf

- 1 1/2 teaspoons Italian seasoning

- 1 teaspoon chili powder

-

2 teaspoons garlic, minced

-

1 pound turkey breast, cooked and diced

-

1/2 pound turkey Italian sausage, cooked, sliced

-

2 onions, sliced

-

1 bell pepper, sliced

-

1/2 teaspoon salt, optional

PREPARATION

1. Combine all ingredients in crockpot. Cover and cook on LOW for 8 to 10 hours.
2. Serves 10 to 12. May be frozen.

Wine-Braised Turkey Breast

INGREDIENTS

- 1 whole boneless turkey breast (about 3 pounds)

- 1 medium onion, halved and thinly sliced

- 1/2 teaspoon thyme

- 1 large clove garlic, thinly sliced

- salt and pepper to taste

- 1/4 cup Madeira wine

- 1 tablespoon honey

- 1 to 2 ounces dried mushrooms, such as Porcini, soaked in 1/4 cup water

- 1 tablespoon cornstarch mixed with with 2 tablespoons cold water

PREPARATION

1. Take turkey breast out of wrapping and netting, and rinse under cold water; pat dry. Place turkey breast in slow cooker; add onion, thyme, garlic, salt & pepper, wine, honey, and mushrooms with soaking liquid. Cover and cook on low for 8 to 10 hours. During the last 30 minutes pour liquid into a container to skim excess fat, if desired, and return broth to pot. Stir cornstarch mixture in and continue cooking until smooth and thickened.
2. Serves 5 to 6.

Apple Betty

INGREDIENTS

- 3 pounds cooking apples, Rome, Granny Smith, Jonathan, etc.

- 10 slices of bread, cubed, about 4 cups of bread cubes

- 1/2 tsp. ground cinnamon

- 1/4 tsp. ground nutmeg

- 1/8 tsp. salt

- 3/4 cup brown sugar, packed

- 1/2 cup melted butter

PREPARATION

1. Wash apples, peel, core, cut into eighths. You should have about 7 to 8 cups of sliced apples. Place apple slices in bottom of buttered crockpot. Combine bread cubes with cinnamon, nutmeg, salt, sugar, butter; toss together. Place on top of apples in crock. Cover and cook on LOW for 2 1/2 to 4 hours.
2. Serves 6.

Apple Butter

INGREDIENTS

-

7 cups applesauce, natural

-

2 cups apple cider

-

1 1/2 cups honey

-

1 tsp ground cinnamon

-

1/4 tsp ground cloves, optional

-

1/2 tsp allspice

PREPARATION

1. In a slow cooker, combine all ingredients. Cover and cook on LOW for 14 to 15 hours or until mixture is a deep brown.
2. Spoon hot apple butter into hot sterilized jars and seal, then process half-pints or pints 10 minutes in a boiling water bath.
3. Makes 4 pints or 8 half-pint jars.

xApple-Coconut Crisp

INGREDIENTS

- 4 large Granny Smith apples, cored, peeled & coarsely chopped (about 4 cups)

- 1/2 cup sweetened flaked coconut

- 1 tablespoon flour

- 1/3 cup brown sugar

- 1/2 cup butterscotch or caramel ice cream topping (fat-free is fine)

- 1/2 teaspoon cinnamon

- 1/3 cup flour

- 1/2 cup quick rolled oats

- 2 tablespoons butter

PREPARATION

1. In a 1 1/2-quart baking dish that fits in the slow cooker/Crock Pot, combine apples with coconut, 1 tablespoon flour, 1/3 cup brown sugar, and cinnamon. Drizzle with the ice cream topping. Combine remaining ingredients in a small bowl with a fork or pastry cutter and sprinkle over apple mixture. Cover and cook on high for 2 1/2 to 3 hours, until apples are tender. Serve warm with vanilla ice cream or whipped topping.

Apple Cranberry Crisp

INGREDIENTS

- 3 large apples, peeled, cored, and sliced

- 1 cup cranberries

- 3/4 cup brown sugar

- 1/3 cup rolled oats (quick cooking)

- 1/4 tsp. salt

- 1 tsp. cinnamon

- 1/3 cup butter, softened

PREPARATION

1. Place apple slices and cranberries in slow cooker. Mix remaining ingredients in a bowl; sprinkle over top of apple and cranberries. Place 4 or 5 paper towels over the top of the slow cooker and place a utensi, such as a wooden spoon over the top to keep cover from sealing tightly. Set cover on top. This allows the steam to escape. Turn slow cooker to high and cook for about 2 hours.
2. Serves 4.

Apple Cranberry Compote

INGREDIENTS

- 6 cooking apples, peeled, cored, and sliced

- 1 cup fresh cranberries

- 1 cup granulated sugar

- 1/2 teaspoon grated orange zest

- 1/2 cup water

- 3 tablespoons port wine or orange juice

- heavy cream, optional

PREPARATION

1. Arrange apple slices and cranberries in slow cooker.
   Sprinkle sugar over fruit. Add orange zest, water and wine.
   Stir to mix ingredients. Cover, cook on LOW for 4 to 6 hours,
   until apples are tender. Serve warm fruits with the juices,
   topped with cream, if desired.
2. Serves 6.

Apple-Date Pudding

INGREDIENTS

- 5 Jonathan or Granny Smith apples, peeled, cored and diced (or other cooking apples)

- 3/4 cup granulated sugar

- 1/2 cup chopped dates

- 1/2 cup toasted, chopped pecans•

- 2 tablespoons flour

- 1 teaspoon baking powder

- 1/8 teaspoon salt

- 1/4 teaspoon nutmeg

- 1/4 teaspoon cinnamon

- 2 tablespoons melted butter

- 1 egg, beaten

PREPARATION

1. In the slow cooker, place apples, sugar, dates and pecans; stir to blend. In a separate bowl, mix together flour, baking powder, salt, nutmeg and cinnamon; stir into apple mixture. Drizzle melted butter over mixture and stir. Stir in beaten egg. Cover and cook on LOW for 3 to 4 hours. Serve warm.
2. •To toast nuts, spread out in a single layer on a baking sheet. Toast in a 350° oven, stirring occasionally, for 10 to 15 minutes.
3. Or, toast in an ungreased skillet over medium heat, stirring, until golden brown and aromatic.

Apple-Nut Cheesecake

INGREDIENTS

●

Crust:

●

1 cup (scant) graham cracker crumbs

●

1/2 teaspoon cinnamon

●

2 tablespoons sugar

●

3 tablespoons butter, melted

●

1/4 cup finely chopped pecans or walnuts

●

Filling:

●

16 ounces cream cheese

●

1/4 cup brown sugar

●

1/2 cup granulated white sugar

●

2 large eggs

●

3 tablespoons heavy whipping cream

- 1 tablespoon cornstarch

- 1 teaspoon vanilla

-

Topping:

- 1 large apple, thinly sliced (about 1 1/2 cups)

- 1 teaspoon cinnamon

- 1/4 cup sugar

- 1 tablespoon finely chopped pecans or walnuts

PREPARATION

1. Combine crust ingredients; pat into a 7-inch springform pan.
2. Beat sugars into cream cheese until smooth and creamy. Beat in eggs, whipping cream, cornstarch, and vanilla. Beat for about 3 minutes on medium speed of a hand-held electric mixer. Pour mixture into the prepared crust.
3. Combine apple slices with sugar, cinnamon and nuts; place topping evenly over the top of cheesecake. Place the cheesecake on a rack (or "ring" of aluminum foil to keep it off the bottom of the pot) in the Crock Pot.
4. Cover and cook on high for 2 1/2 to 3 hours.
5. Let stand in the covered pot (after turning it off) for about 1 to 2 hours, until cool enough to handle.
6. Cool thoroughly before removing pan sides.
7. Chill before serving; store leftovers in the refrigerator.
8. Oven: Bake at 325° F about 45 minutes to 1 hour, then turn the oven off and let it cool in the oven for about 4 hours.

Apple Pie Coffee Cake

INGREDIENTS

-

Apple Mixture:

-

1 can (20 oz) apple pie filling, apple slices broken up somewhat

-

1/2 teaspoon cinnamon

-

3 tablespoons brown sugar

-

.

-

Cake Batter:

-

2 small yellow cake mixes (Jiffy - 9-ounce each)

-

2 eggs, beaten

-

1/2 cup sour cream (light)

-

3 tablespoons softened butter or margarine

-

1/2 cup evaporated milk

-

1/2 teaspoon cinnamon

•

1 teaspoon butter or margarine for greasing slow cooker

PREPARATION

1. Combine ingredients for apple mixture in a small bowl. Combine batter ingredients; mix well. Generouslly butter the sides and bottom of a 3 1/2 quart slow cooker/Crock Pot. Spread about half the apple mixture in the bottom of the pot. Spoon 1/2 the batter over the apple mixture. Spoon the remaining apple mixture over the batter, then cover with remaining batter. Cover and cook on high for 2 to 2 1/2 hours.

2. Turn heat off, leave cover ajar slightly, and cool for about 15 minutes. Invert on a plate, retrieving any apples left in the bottom of the pot and placing on top of the cake. Makes a cake about 7 inches in diameter and 3 1/2-inches high.

Variations:

1. Substitute peach or other pie filling

3. Add chopped pecans or walnuts to the apple mixture

Apple Pudding Cake

INGREDIENTS

- 2 cups granulated sugar

- 1 cup vegetable oil

- 2 eggs

- 2 teaspoons vanilla extract

- 2 cups all-purpose flour

- 1 teaspoon baking soda

- 1 teaspoon nutmeg

- 2 cups cooking apples, unpeeled, cored, finely chopped

- 1 cup chopped walnuts

PREPARATION

1. In a large mixer bowl, beat together the sugar, oil, eggs, and vanilla. Add flour, soda, and nutmeg; mix well.
2. Spray a two-pound can with cooking spray or grease and flour it well, or use another baking dish which will fit in your slow cooker.
3. Pour batter into can or baking dish, filling up to 2/3 full.
4. Place it in Crock-Pot or slow cooker. Do not add water to the pot.
5. Cover but leave cover slightly ajar to let steam escape.
6. Cook on high 3 1/2 to 4 hours. Don't peek before the last hour of baking.
7. Cake is done when top is set.
8. Let stand in can a few minutes before tipping it out onto a plate. Serve with whipped topping, sweetened whipped cream, or a Dessert Sauce.

Apricot Nut Bread

INGREDIENTS

- 3/4 cup dried apricots

- 1 cup flour

- 2 tsp baking powder

- 1/4 tsp baking soda

- 1/2 tsp salt

- 1/2 cup granulated sugar

- 1/2 cup whole wheat flour

- 3/4 cup milk

- 1 egg, slightly beaten

- 1 Tbsp grated orange rind

- 1 Tbsp vegetable oil

- 1 cup coarsely chopped pecans

PREPARATION

1. Place the apricots on a cutting board and sprinkle 1 tablespoon of flour over them. Dip a knife into the flour and chop the dried apricots finely. Flour the knife often to keep the apricots from sticking together. Sift together the remaining flour, baking powder, baking soda, salt, and sugar into a large mixing bowl. Stir in the whole wheat flour. Combine the milk, egg, orange rind, and oil. Stir into the flour mixture.

2. Fold in the cut up apricots, any flour left on the cutting board, and the chopped pecans. Pour into a well greased, floured baking unit or other heat-proof baking dish or casserole which fits in your slow cooker. Cover and place on a rack (or crumpled foil) in the slow cooker, but prop the lid open a fraction with a twist of foil to let excess steam escape. Cook apricot nut bread on High for 4 to 6 hours. Cool on a rack for 10 minutes. Serve warm or cold.

3. Makes 4 to 6 servings.

Baked Apples

INGREDIENTS

- 6 large cooking apples

- 3/4 cup orange juice

- 2 teaspoons grated orange peel

- 1 teaspoon grated lemon peel

- 3/4 cup blush wine or cranberry-apple juice

- 1/4 teaspoon cinnamon

- 1/2 cup light brown sugar

- whipped cream

PREPARATION

1. Remove cores from apples and place in slow cooker. In a small bowl, combine orange juice, grated orange peel, grated lemon peel, wine or juice, cinnamon, and brown sugar. Pour over apples. Cover crockpot and cook on low for about 3 1/2 hours, or until apples are tender. Cool slightly and serve with whipped cream or whipped topping.

Baked Apples II

INGREDIENTS

- 6 to 8 medium cooking apples (McIntosh, Rome Beauty, Granny Smith, Fuji, Jonathan, etc.)

- 2 to 3 tablespoons raisins

- 1/4 cup granulated sugar

- 1 teaspoon cinnamon, divided

- 2 tablespoons butter, cut in small pieces

PREPARATION

1. Remove a little of the peel around the top of the apples and remove the cores.
2. In a bowl, mix raisins, sugar, and 1/2 teaspoon cinnamon; fill center of apples.
3. Place the apples in the slow cooker and sprinkle with the remaining cinnamon. Dot with the butter pieces.
4. Pour 1/2 cup warm water around the apples.
5. Cover and cook on LOW for 6 to 8 hours, until apples are tender.

Baked Custard

INGREDIENTS

- 3 eggs, lightly beaten

- 1/3 cup granulated sugar

- 1 teaspoon vanilla

- 2 cups milk

- 1/4 teaspoon ground nutmeg

PREPARATION

1. In a mixing bowl combine eggs, sugar, vanilla and milk; mix well. Pour into a lightly buttered 1- or 1 1/2-quart baking dish or souffle which will fit in the slow cooker, and sprinkle with the nutmeg. Place a rack or ring of aluminum foil in the slow cooker, then add 1 1/2 to 2 cups of hot water to the pot. Cover the baking dish with aluminum foil and place on the rack in the crockpot. Cover and cook on high for 2 1/2 to 3 hours, or until set.
2. Serves 4 to 6.

Banana Bread

INGREDIENTS

- 1/3 cup shortening

- 1/2 cup sugar

- 2 eggs

- 1 3/4 cups flour

- 1 tsp baking powder

- 1/2 tsp salt

- 1/2 tsp baking soda

- 1 cup mashed bananas

- 1/2 cup raisins or chopped dates

- 1/2 cup chopped pecans, optional

PREPARATION

1. In mixing bowl, cream together shortening and sugar; add eggs and beat well. Add dry ingredients alternately with mashed banana; stir in raisins or chopped dates and chopped pecans, if using. Grease a 4-cup can and pour batter in it. Cover top of can with 6 to 8 layers of paper towel; and place on rack in cooker. Cover crockpot and cook on HIGH for 2 to 3 hours (or until bread is done). Shared on the forum.

Banana Nut Bread

INGREDIENTS

- 1 cup butter or margarine

- 2 cups sugar

- 4 eggs

- 1/4 teaspoon salt

- 2 teaspoons soda

- 4 cups flour

- 6 large bananas, very ripe, mashed

- 1 cup finely chopped pecans

PREPARATION

1. Cream together butter and sugar. Add eggs, one at a time, beating after each addition. Sift dry ingredients together; add to creamed mixture. Stir in bananas and chopped pecans.
2. Pour banana nut bread batter into 2 well greased loaf pans; bake at 325° for about 1 hour and 15 minutes, or until a toothpick inserted in center comes out clean. This banana nut bread recipe makes 2 loaves.

Candied Bananas

INGREDIENTS

- 6 ripe but firm bananas, peeled

- 1/2 cup flaked coconut

- 1/2 tsp ground cinnamon

- 1/4 tsp salt

- 1/2 cup dark corn syrup

- 1/4 cup butter, melted

- 1 tablespoon grated lemon peel

- 3 to 4 tablespoons lemon juice (1 medium lemon)

PREPARATION

1. Arrange peeled bananas in the bottom of crockpot; sprinkle with coconut, cinnamon, and the salt.
2. Combine dark corn syrup, butter, lemon peel and juice; pour over banana layer.
3. Cover and cook on LOW for 1 1/2 to 2 hours.

Carmel Apples

INGREDIENTS

- 2 packages (14oz each) caramels

- 1/4 cup water

- 8 medium apples, such as McIntosh, Gala, or Fuji

- sticks for apples

PREPARATION

1. In slow cooker, combine caramels and water. Cover and cook on high for 1 to 1 1/2 hours, or until caramels are melted, stirring frequently.
2. Meanwhile, line a baking pan with wax paper; butter the paper.
3. Wash and dry the apples. Insert a stick into stem end of each apple. Reduce crockpot heat to LOW.
4. **Note:** If the caramel does happen to scorch, put it through a mesh strainer and discard any dark particles.
5. Put the sauce into a saucepan or back into the cleaned slow cooker and keep warm while you dip the apples.
6. Dip apple into hot caramel; turn to coat entire surface. Holding apple above pot, scrape off excess accumulation of caramel from bottom apple.

7. Place coated apples on prepared wax paper in pan. As you near the bottom of the pot, use a spoon to spoon hot caramel over apples. Put the pan of coated apples in the refrigerator to set thoroughly. Use caution if children are helping; the crockpot will probably be quite hot to the touch and the caramel could scald.
8. Makes 8 caramel apples.

Caramel Rum Fondue

INGREDIENTS

- 1 bag (14 ounces) ounces caramels

- 2/3 cup heavy cream or whipping cream

- 1/2 cup miniature marshmallows

- 2 to 3 teaspoons rum or 1/2 teaspoon rum extract

PREPARATION

1. Combine caramels and whipping cream in slow cooker. Cover and cook on LOW until the caramels have melted, about 1 1/2 hours. Stir in marshmallows and rum flavoring until well blended. Cover and continue cooking for about 30 minutes longer.
2. Serve with apple wedges, pound cake cubes, or use as a sauce for gingerbread or ice cream.

Cherry Crisp

INGREDIENTS

- 1 can (21 oz) cherry pie filling

- 2/3 cup brown sugar

- 1/2 cup quick-cooking oats

- 1/2 cup flour

- 1 teaspoon vanilla

- 1/3 cup butter, softened

PREPARATION

1. Lightly butter a 3 1/2-quart slow cooker/Crock Pot. Place cherry pie filling in the slow cooker/Crock Pot. Combine dry ingredients with vanilla and mix well; cut in butter with a pastry cutter or fork. Sprinkle crumbs over the cherry pie filling. Cook for 5 hours on low.

Chocolate Clusters

INGREDIENTS

- 2 pounds white almond bark or white chocolate for dipping

- 4 ounces German's sweet chocolate or milk chocolate for dipping

- 1 package semisweet chocolate chips (12 ounces)

- 24 ounces dry roasted peanuts

PREPARATION

1. Put all ingredients in crockpot; cover and cook on high for 1 hour. Do not stir. Turn Crock Pot to low and stir every 15 minutes for 1 hour longer. Drop on waxed paper and let cool. Store candy in a tightly covered container.

CPSIA information can be obtained
at www.ICGtesting.com
Printed in the USA
BVHW091017190421
605287BV00002B/191

9 781801 987332